VORTEX CONTROL SELF-DEFENSE

HAND-TO-HAND STREET FIGHTING TACTICS

SAM FURY

Illustrated by
NEIL GERMIO

Copyright SF Nonfiction Books © 2017

www.SFNonfictionBooks.com

All Rights Reserved
No part of this document may be reproduced without written consent from the author.

This publication has the approval of Peter Sunbye, creator of Vortex Control Self-Defense.

WARNINGS AND DISCLAIMERS

The information in this publication is made public for reference only.

Neither the author, publisher, nor anyone else involved in the production of this publication is responsible for how the reader uses the information or the result of his/her actions.

CONTENTS

Introduction   vii

Explanation of Terms   1
Principles of Self-Defense   3
Stepping   15
Weight Distribution Drill   17
Bombs   19
Bouncing Kicks   23

ENTRIES

Slap Entries   27
Thrust Entries   34
Curve Entries   37
Contact Entries   40
Rib Entries   42

Hand Formula   44
Lock Flow Drill   49
References   68

Author Recommendations   69
About Sam Fury   71

THANKS FOR YOUR PURCHASE

Did you know you can get FREE chapters of any SF Nonfiction Book you want?

https://offers.SFNonfictionBooks.com/Free-Chapters

You will also be among the first to know of FREE review copies, discount offers, bonus content, and more.

Go to:

https://offers.SFNonfictionBooks.com/Free-Chapters

Thanks again for your support.

INTRODUCTION

In this self-defense training manual, Sam Fury puts Vortex Control Self-Defense lessons learned in the Philippines onto paper.

Vortex Control Self-Defense is a unique fighting system created by Peter Sunbye. To create this system of self-defense, Peter traveled for 20+ years, searching for "lost" self-defense techniques.

He combined a number of martial arts, including GM Lawrence Lee's Tong Kune Do kung fu, Wing Chun, Balintawak Arnis Escrima, and Panatukan to create a highly effective and relatively easy to learn self-defense system. Once the basics are learned, Vortex Control Self-Defense can be applied effectively by almost anyone, regardless of their dexterity, strength, or fitness level.

This volume covers hand-to-hand combat and has been written under the approval of Peter Sunbye.

EXPLANATION OF TERMS

A few terms are used throughout this book to help describe the flow of movement.

Lead/Rear Side

Your lead side is whichever side of your body is forward-most and your rear side is whichever side of your body is rear-most. For example, if you're in a right-foot-forward stance, then your right side is your lead side, and your left side is your rear side.

Inside/Outside of Your Opponent's Guard

When your opponent's guard is up, you can place your arm either inside or outside of it.

Being inside your opponent's guard means that your limb is in between his limbs, closer to his center. Your arm is sandwiched by his.

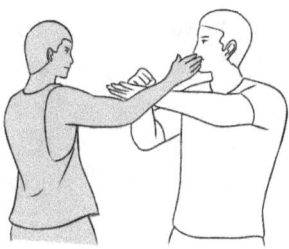

Being outside your opponent's guard means your opponent's limbs are both to either the left or right of your limb.

The pictures demonstrate being inside/outside of your opponent's guard with your arms, but it also applies to your legs. That is, you need to step to the outside of your opponent's guard in order to get behind him.

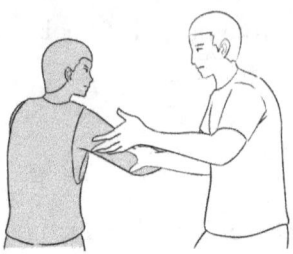

Just as you can be inside or outside your opponent's guard, he can be inside/outside yours.

Guarding Your Opponent's Limb

The expression "to guard your opponent's limb" means to put your limb close or on his limb so that you can't be struck by it. It is a pre-emptive defensive maneuver that may also be referred to as "covering your opponent's limb."

Throughout this book, the word "limb" is replaced as appropriate. For example, in the previous picture the man is using his right hand to guard/cover the woman's right elbow.

PRINCIPLES OF SELF-DEFENSE

The following principles are the core of Vortex Control Self-Defense. Although explained in reference to hand-to-hand combat, they are also applicable to weaponry.

Without these principles, the rest of this book is just a bunch of techniques that you can mimic. With them, the techniques in this book become a collection of examples of how the principles can be applied. You can then replicate techniques and/or create customized to ones.

The Vortex Control Self-Defense principles are all of equal importance, and are presented here in alphabetical order.

Constant Barrage

In Vortex Control Self-Defense there, you are constantly slapping, twisting, pulling, and pushing your opponent. This serves at least one (and usually several, if not all) of the following purposes:

- It confuses and disorients your opponent.
- It often lets you move your opponent one way while striking from the opposite direction. This increases the force of your strike.
- The movements in themselves bring a certain degree of discomfort and pain.
- It lets you place your opponent in the ideal position for your next move.

This also makes use of Newton's first law of motion, which states that:

> "An object at rest stays at rest, and an object in motion stays in motion with the same speed and in the same direction unless acted upon by an unbalanced force."

In reference to your movement, this means that it's better for you to keep moving once you're in motion. This is because it takes more energy to stop and restart than it does to continue an existing motion. In addition, the continued motion will be faster and therefore more powerful than if you were to start from inertia.

Counters

In martial arts, a counter is an attack made in response to your opponent's attack. It is about being proactive.

There is always a counter to your opponent's move, and there is a counter to your counter, and a counter to that counter. It can go on forever. The victor will be whoever has the foresight and/or intuition to out-counter their opponent.

Close combat is a game of chess. Fast chess. Instinctive chess.

Note: The closer you get to your opponent, the fewer opportunities there are for counters. You can use this to your advantage by first closing distance while gaining an advantageous position, and then finishing the fight before your opponent recovers.

Grounding

Grounding yourself means being in solid contact with the ground.

When you're grounded, you have more stability, and can therefore generate more powerful attacks. Power in strikes comes up from the ground. This is a well-known concept in the world of martial arts.

A simple exercise you can do to get the feeling of grounding is to pretend that you're drilling your body into the ground.

Grounding in this way is also well demonstrated in the weight distribution drill.

The act of grounding can also be used to increase damage by letting gravity do the work. This is well demonstrated in angulated stepping and the bomb-kick.

To get the feeling of using grounding in this manner, lift both your legs off the ground without jumping. Just let gravity do its thing.

Fulcrums

Body mechanics, paired with physics, play a big part in the efficiency of Vortex Control Self-Defense. By using parts of your body as fulcrums, you can gain more leverage, apply locks, break limbs, etc.

One-Handed Fighting

Both arms are used in the demonstrations in this book, but the unarmed portion of Vortex Control Self-Defense is developed so that most of the techniques can be done one-handed. This becomes extremely useful in real-life scenarios, such as when you are holding something you can't drop, like a baby, or when your arm gets injured. Once you have a good grasp of the techniques, you should train to do them with one hand. Just don't use your rear hand.

Power Angles

This is another principle based on physics and body mechanics.

There are certain angles that create the strongest frames. Your limbs should never be below 120° or above 160°.

120° is best for defense. Any smaller of an angle, and your arm will easily collapse when it's pushed towards you.

160° is best for attack. Any larger of an angle, and your arm can be easily pushed to the side. Holding it at an angle greater than 160° will also make it more susceptible to being captured—by being placed in a lock, for example.

As a rule, keep your limb at 120°. When you strike, extend it to 160° and then let your body push through. This combines power angles with grounding. Add in spring-loading and aim for the spine and you have the ideal the Vortex Control Self-Defense strike.

Spine Center

The Spine Center principle is based on the centerline theory, which is common in many martial arts, including Wing Chun. To explain the concept, here is an excerpt from the book *Basic Wing Chun Training* by Sam Fury:

www.SFNonfictionBooks.com/Basic-Wing-Chun-Training

Your centerline is an imaginary line drawn vertically down the center of your body. All the vital organs are located near the center of the body. Keep it away from your opponent by angling it away from him/her.

Controlling the position of your centerline in relation to your opponent's is done with footwork. Understanding the centerline will allow you to instinctively know where your opponent is.

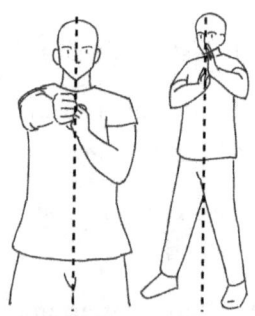

Your central line (different from your centerline) is drawn from your angled center to your opponent.

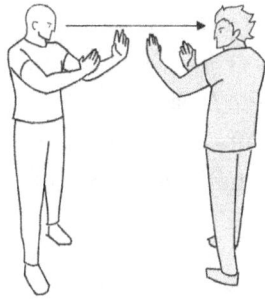

Offensively, you generate the most power when punching out from your center, since you can incorporate your whole body and hips.

When you're attacking in a straight line, your centerline should face away from your opponent, while your central line faces his/her center.

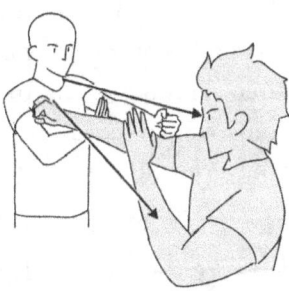

With hook punches and other circular attacks, the center- and central lines merge.

There are three main guidelines for the centerline.

- The one who controls the centerline will control the fight.
- Protect and maintain your own centerline while you control and exploit your opponent's.
- Control the centerline by occupying it.

In Vortex Control Self-Defense, instead of putting your offensive focus on your opponent's centerline as described above, focus on his spine. Doing so makes the idea of striking through your target more intuitive. An added advantage is that his spine can be affected by the many jerks, twists, etc. that are commonly used in Vortex Control Self-Defense.

Spring-Loading

Yet another principle based on the combination of body mechanics and physics is spring-loading.

The basic premise is that your muscles can be pushed in like a spring. These springs are then released in strikes, increasing speed and therefore power.

Speed in strikes is not just about how fast you reach the target. You must also be quick to recover. Recovery is the process of reloading the spring, which you can then send out again. In your arm, your triceps are the spring forward and your biceps are the spring back. Alternating spring-loading your arms allows you to make multiple strikes in very quick succession.

You can and should also spring-load your legs. The groin kick is a clear demonstration of this, but the motion should be present in all your movements.

It's important to remain relaxed. The spring is loaded and released, but never tensed so much that it slows you down.

Taking Space

Always crowd your opponent. Get in his space and claim it. Constantly push him back, and don't let up. This will unbalance him both mentally and physically.

Following the Thank You Principle

Take whatever your opponent gives you and use it to your advantage. If he applies pressure in a particular direction, flow with it. Redirect it if needed, but don't directly oppose it.

Those that want to become really good at this are encouraged to practice Chi Sao. Although live instruction is always preferred, the book *How to do Chi Sao* by Sam Fury is highly recommended.

www.SFNonfictionBooks.com/Chi-Sao

Another use of the thank you principle is to always take something back. For example, when retracting your limb from a strike, grab your opponent's arm or nose-ring.

Vibrating

In Vortex Control Self-Defense, the principle of vibrating is used to enhance the effectiveness of movement. It can be applied in many situations, such as when you're increasing the force in locks, making repetitive strikes, escaping holds, etc.

The following examples offer safe demonstrations of the effectiveness of vibrating:

The first example is a shirt-grab escape. Say an attacker grabs you by the shirt-front. Reach over his arms and grab his right wrist. At the same time, use your left hand to grab the same arm.

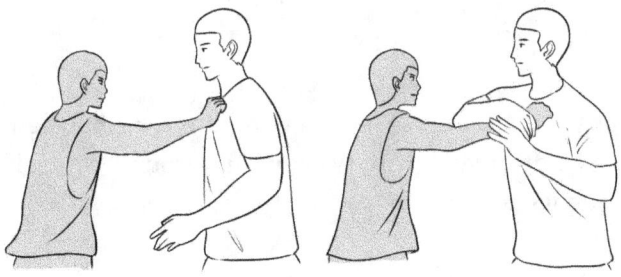

To release your opponent's grip, twist your body to your right using a waterfall motion.

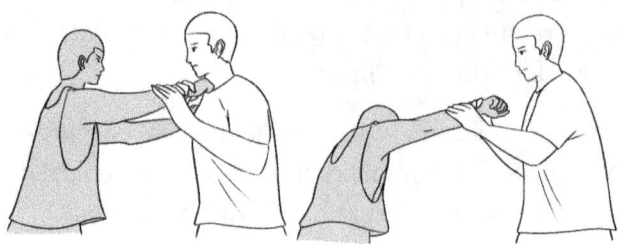

This move itself is a common and effective self-defense technique, but when your attacker is much stronger than you, it may not work. Increase its effectiveness by vibrating.

As you twist your body, make small, fast, jerking movements. Concentrate these movements into your twisting motion, especially where your opponent is gripping you.

The next example is a rear bear hug escape. Say an attacker puts you in a rear bear hug with your arms pinned. A common way to get out of this is with rear elbows, but if your opponent's grip is too tight, you won't have the room to do this. Vibrate your body to create space.

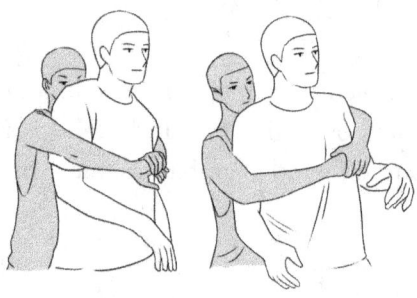

As soon as you have even just enough room, rear elbow left and then right. Finally, drop your body weight and ground yourself to break your opponent's grip.

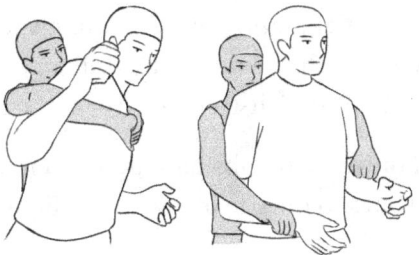

Vortex

By using the motion of a vortex (like water going down a sinkhole) you can easily break through your opponent's defense. For example, if your opponent is pushing your hand in a certain direction, you can use a vortex motion to move under and around it. This is actually the basis of the curve entry.

Another way to use the vortex is if your opponent grabs your arm. A fast vortex motion will most likely free you from his grip while you counter-strike in the same motion. In most cases, you'll want to vortex towards your opponent's spine.

Warfare Strategy

The strategy for attack in Vortex Control Self-Defense mimics that of warfare.

Intelligence. First, you must gather intelligence so you can make the right decision regarding your enemy. In warfare, this is done through methods such as espionage. In self-defense, it's better understood as "sizing up" your opponent.

Within a few seconds of studying your enemy, you can determine any weaknesses he has (such as obvious injuries), sense his fear (or lack thereof), assess his ability (speed, strength, skill), etc. You can also assess your surroundings and identify possible escape routes, available weapons, etc.

Bombs. After your initial assessment, assuming you feel that fighting is necessary, attack with bombs. The military uses planes and mortars. In Vortex Control Self-Defense, we use bomb-kicks.

Infantry. Finally, once the bombs have done their job, the infantry is sent in. This translates to the use of entry techniques and the fighting formula.

Waterfall

The analogy of water going over the edge of a waterfall is often used to explain how to perform certain movements used in the techniques. The free-fall of water is also akin to grounding. Combing the three actions of waterfall, grounding, and vortex is extremely powerful.

Weaponizing

The principle of weaponizing means to make as many of your movements as much like attacks as possible, even if they are primarily defensive or neutral. Here are some examples:

- Instead of just placing your foot down after a kick, stomp your opponent's knee or foot.
- When defending against an incoming strike, don't just block it. Instead, block it in a way that hurts your opponent as well. Punch his arm (a stop-hit), for example.
- Your intention may be to apply a lock, but you can make various strikes in the process.
- After hitting your opponent, hit him again while retracting your limb.

Yin and Yang

The well-known Chinese Taoism concept of yin and yang is also applied in Vortex Control Self-Defense, where yin is "soft" and yang is "hard."

Soft does not equal weak, and it is the combination of soft and hard, fast and slow, light and heavy (grounded), etc. that will make your techniques work together.

Here are some examples to demonstrate the use of yin and yang in the context of Vortex Control Self-Defense. These are just a few examples of a concept that applies to everything in the universe.

- Tai Chi is very yin (slow and soft) in practice, and to the layman it may seem useless for combat, but if you speed the movements up to become yang (hard and fast), they can be devastating.
- In training, it's useful to use more yin and less yang. Doing things slowly (yin) first allows your mind and body to "soak in" the lessons. If you go straight to yang, not only will you learn poor technique, but your chances of injury while training will also be much higher.
- When an opponent strikes, you can receive his attack using yin, going with the flow of his motion. You may also defend against it using yang, attacking your opponent's limb as he strikes. A third option is to use a combination of yin and yang, where you receive the attack by flowing with it and then redirect the energy to counterattack.
- When you're using your hand to meet an attack, if your fingers face forward, it is considered yin. If your fingers face up, it's Yang. When your fingers are up, the hard, bony part of your hand is exposed, but when your fingers are forward it's not.

Related Chapters:

- Stepping
- Bombs
- Weight Distribution Drill
- Curve Entries
- Bouncing Kicks

STEPPING

Spring Semi-Forward Stepping

Spring semi-forward stepping is used to close distance.

In this movement, your back heel is up. This turns your calf muscle into a double spring—one behind your knee and one at your heel. Releasing these springs propels your whole body forward.

Take a small step forward with your lead foot and move your rear foot into the original position of your lead. Your stance should never be too exaggerated.

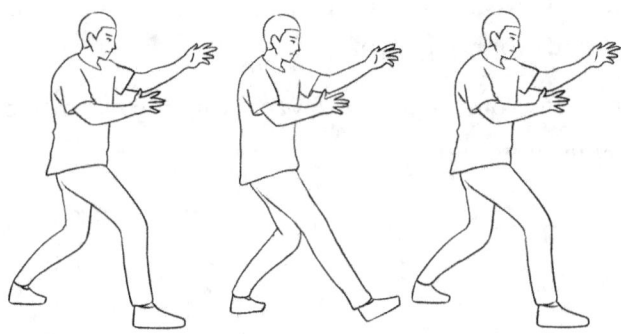

Keep most of your weight on your rear leg. The heel of your front foot should land first, followed by the toes of both feet. This will keep you well-grounded and ready for the next move.

When using the spring semi-forward step, you'll most likely be attacking, which means your attacking arm (usually your lead) will be at 160°, but never more.

Remember that 120° is the strongest angle for defense, and 160° is the best for offense. Never go outside of these angles.

Angulated Stepping

With this method of stepping, you close in on your opponent by going around him/her first. This allows you to:

1. Maneuver around any linear attacks.
2. Collect bodyweight to put more power behind your strike by grounding yourself.

To practice angulated stepping, start in a neutral position. Step towards your opponent, but at an angle. Always point your extremities towards your opponent—it will focus your power.

Change the direction of your toes to face your opponent. Put all your weight onto your lead foot and then step through with your rear leg, directly towards your opponent.

You'll "fall" into your opponent's space, which will put more bodyweight behind your blow.

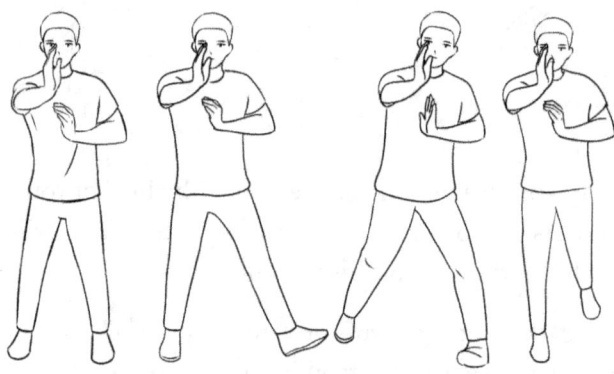

WEIGHT DISTRIBUTION DRILL

This drill trains your body to put weight behind your strikes. Start in a neutral stance, with your left hand up in a guard position.

Shift your weight onto your right leg as you turn your body to the right. Your left arm should come down as your waist moves, following the movement of your waist naturally manner. That is, your arm should move because of your waist motion.

Bring yourself back to a neutral position. Mimic defense with your left hand, using a 120° angle. Continue to turn to your left. Follow the movement of your waist with your right arm for a big hit.

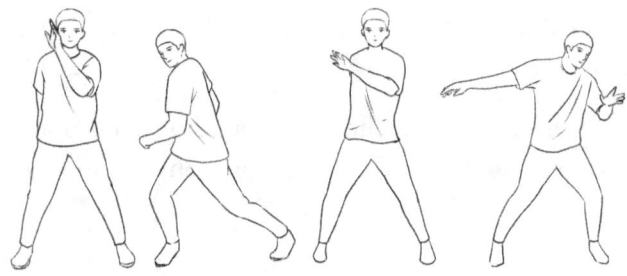

As you drop your weight onto your left leg, hook your right arm in to hit your opponent. Repeat the action from left to right, and so on.

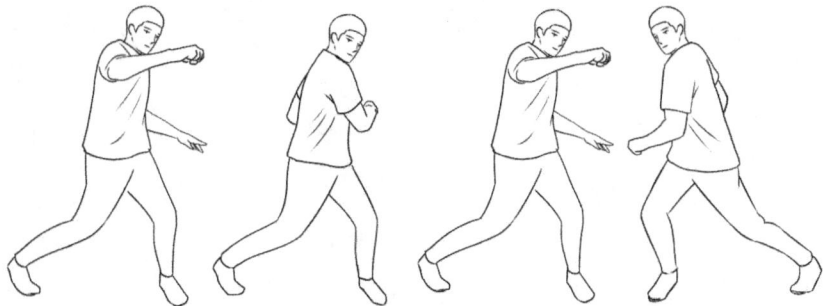

The above demonstrates big circular hitting, but the drill can also be applied to linear strikes.

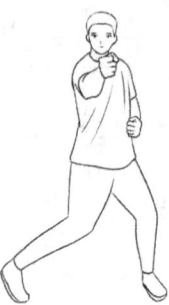

Whichever leg you're placing your weight on can be considered your brake. It grounds you. If you don't do this, you'll lose balance. At the end of the hit, that same leg then becomes the spring to accelerate the circular movement.

Once you're used to the feeling of grounding (and you can do it without losing your balance), concentrate on keeping relaxed and flowing.

BOMBS

Bombs are your first line of defense and offense. There are four of them.

Defensive Bomb

The defensive bomb is used for short-range defense. This move is used when you've been caught off-guard, so it's likely your hands will be down at the time. It's a "panic" move.

As soon as you notice the incoming attack, condense yourself down and in. Lower your weight to set a spring. This compression will also ground you, making you more stable. Explode out at your opponent. Put your head back and bring your lead knee up to face him/her. The motion should continue with you bringing your hands out into the ideal defensive angle of 120°.

In this move, your knee is weaponized. It can be used as usual or in a bomb-kick, crushing your opponent's leg (aim for his/her knee). Once you land, you "go to work" on your opponent with entries and follow-ups.

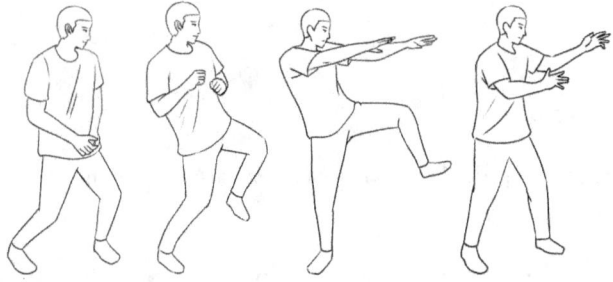

Bomb-Kick

The bomb-kick can be used with any of the bomb techniques. Its power is created by gravity and the "spring" in your leg muscles. You don't put any effort trying to kick through your target. Instead, position your knee as a defensive-aggressive weapon and then release the spring.

When you raise your leg in any of the bombs, ensure your knee comes up pointing towards your opponent. If it's to the side it can be easily pushed away.

Have your foot close to your bum. This "spring-loads" your leg. When you're ready, release the spring so your knee's angle is at 160°. Keep the 160° strong and then allow your body weight to push your foot through your opponent's leg. His/her knee is an ideal target.

A simple exercise you can do is to hold your leg in the "loaded" position and then let it "fire." The aim is to get a feel for stopping at the ideal 160° angle.

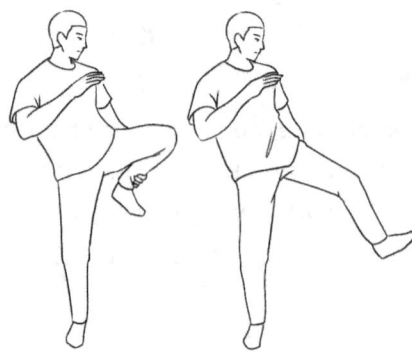

Hammer Bomb

The hammer bomb is a short-range attack. It is dynamic and explosive.

Bring your knee up facing your opponent and attack with your lead hand, using a hammer fist in the over-and-down waterfall action. This allows your arm to come over your opponent's limbs and onto his/her head and/or arms.

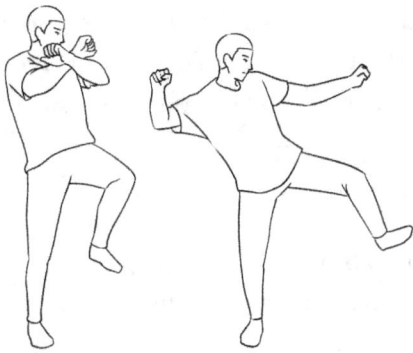

Pendulum Bomb

The pendulum bomb is a long-range attack. It's used when you decide to take someone on before they are close enough to become an immediate threat. Like a pendulum (hence the name) you rock your body back and forth.

First, present your opponent with a long-range weapon (your lead hand) as a feint. You want your opponent to think your hand is your attack, and perhaps even go for your head as a target.

Extend your rear limbs behind you to allow for more reach. As your opponent comes in, draw yourself back in and shift your weight to your rear foot.

Bring your lead knee up and weaponize it into a kick/stomp to your opponent's knee. Guard your head with your rear hand, although it (your head) will most likely be well out of range.

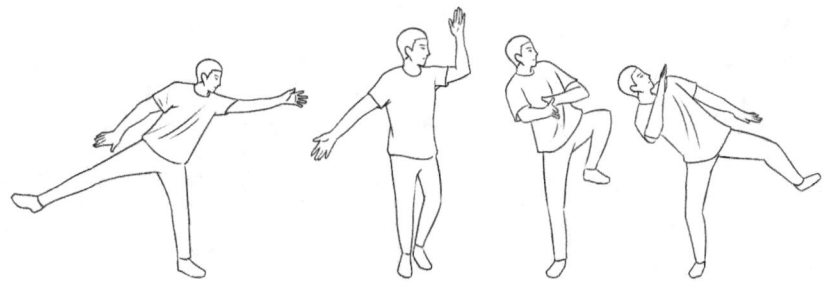

"Fall" forward to drive your foot through your opponent's knee. If you miss your target, then at least you'll be in position to take up your fighting stance, from which you can progress into more attacks.

Cross-Step Bomb

The cross-step bomb is a really long-range attack. It will cover about two feet more ground than the pendulum bomb.

Starting in a right lead stance, bring your left leg forward to cross behind your right. Your left foot should be angled to your rear. Put your weight on your left foot and bring your right knee up facing your opponent.

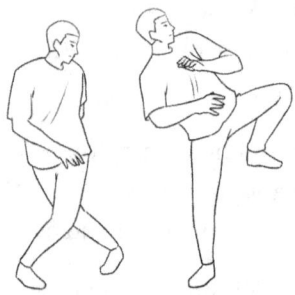

Extend your right foot to the optimal 160°. Fall into it, preferably with your foot crushing through your opponent's knee.

Take up your fighting stance and attack if needed.

BOUNCING KICKS

Groin Kick

After you do a bomb, with or without the follow-through bomb-kick, instead of grounding your lead foot you can bounce it back up for a kick into your opponent's groin.

Do your bomb and then allow your lead foot to fall to the ground, but keep your weight on your rear leg. Bounce your foot back up into your opponent's groin.

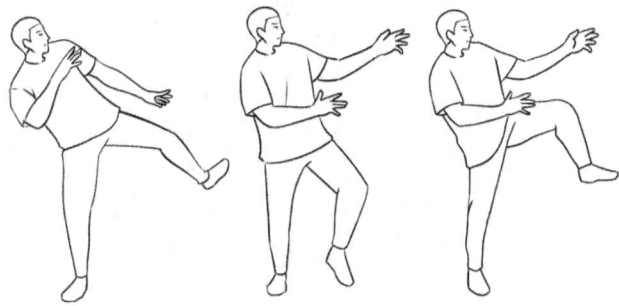

To practice this action, it may help to pretend your knee is like a basketball or yoyo.

Donkey Kick

It may be that you land behind your opponent after your bomb, or that someone approaches you from behind. In this case, you can use a donkey kick.

The same bouncing movement is used, but it's your heel that meets the target.

A variation of the donkey kick is to bring your foot straight up your back into your opponent's jaw. This can be useful if someone puts pressure on you from behind and you're forced to lean forward.

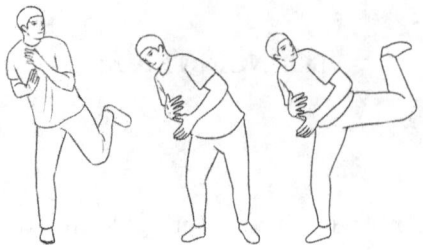

Turning Arm Strike

Another useful strike when someone forces you to lean forward is the turning arm strike.

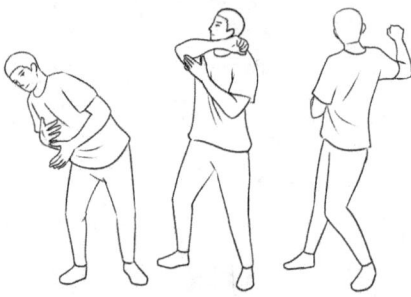

The striking point could be your elbow, forearm, hammer fist, etc.

ENTRIES

An entry technique is used to break through your opponent's initial guard. All the entry techniques described will take you up to the checkmate position.

The following picture illustrates the checkmate position. The main thing is that your arm should be on the outside of your opponent's guard.

Ideally, your arm will be tight against your opponent's. It's also preferable for you to use your non-striking hand to secure your opponent's arm—by grabbing his/her wrist, for example.

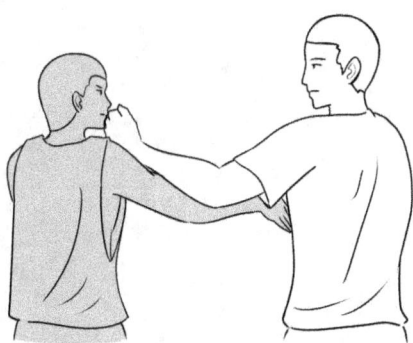

When adopting the checkmate position you may feel more comfortable stepping in, or perhaps stepping through (changing your lead).

The demonstrations show the entry using two hands. They can also be done one-handed. This is something you should experiment with during training.

All entries can be done with an almost simultaneous low kick, which will help confuse your opponent.

Techniques for getting from the entry to the checkmate position are not set in stone. A variety of ways have been demonstrated; these can be mixed and matched to get something that works best for you in a given situation. You should experiment with different starting positions so you can become aware of which entries work best for you in which circumstances.

Related Chapters:

- Stepping

SLAP ENTRIES

Slap entries are ideal to use when your opponent's guard is held out more than 160°, but they can also be used when your opponent's guard is within the power angles (120° to 160°). The basis of the slap entry is to knock your opponent's hand horizontally to clear a path for your attack. Often, the initial slap is a distraction technique. It's subtle, but helps to confuse your opponent.

Outside Parry Entry

Step in and use your lead hand to lightly tap and bounce off your opponent's extended arm at his/her wrist. Almost simultaneously, follow your lead hand with your rear to guide your opponent's arm to the outside so you command the centerline.

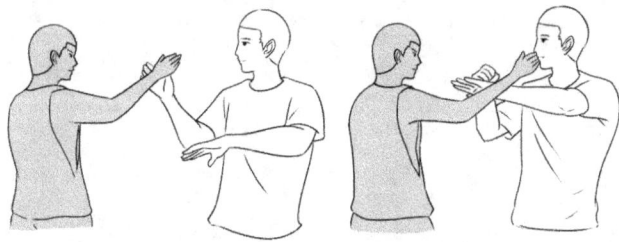

Strike your opponent with your lead as soon as your opponent's centerline is cleared. Next, cross your lead hand over to keep your opponent's lead under control while you strike with your rear.

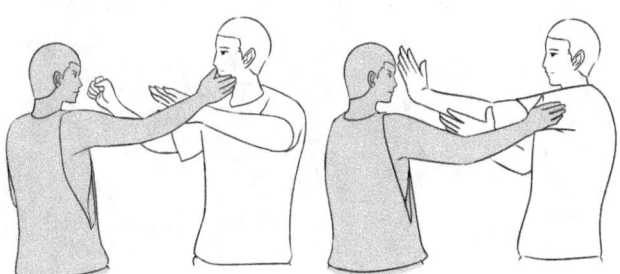

Use your right hand to guide your opponent's lead arm across his/her body. Strike your opponent's ribs. Notice the pointed knuckle fist in the image below, which is used to dig in between the ribs. A normal fist will also suffice.

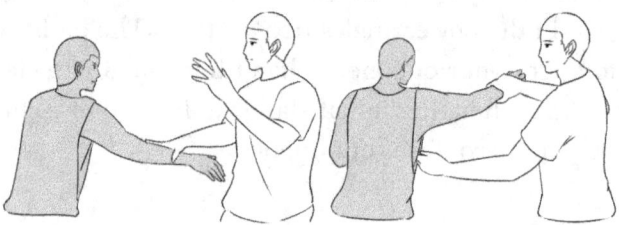

Without letting go of your opponent's wrist, adopt the checkmate position.

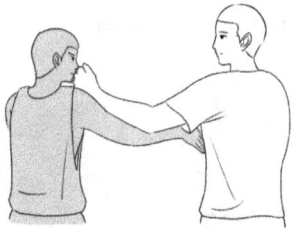

Inside Parry Entry

Use your lead hand to tap and bounce off your opponent's lead. Almost simultaneously, use your rear hand to slap your opponent's hand back to the inside of his/her body. Strike with your lead.

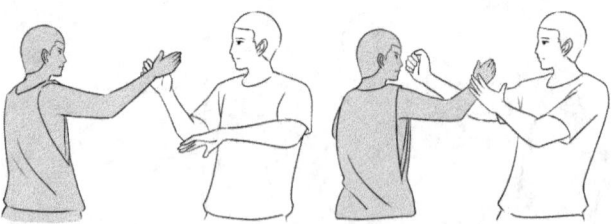

Bring your lead hand straight back and collect your opponent's lead hand on the way as you adopt the checkmate position.

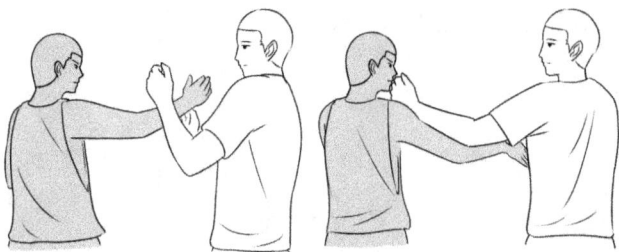

Flick Entry

With your lead hand, slap through your opponent's lower arm and bring it to your centerline.

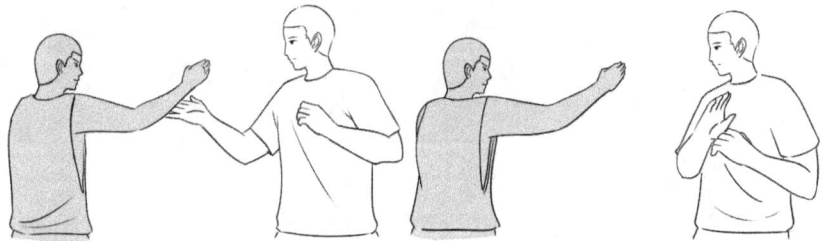

As you step forward, press you rear hand against your opponent's lead arm, just enough to clear the centerline so your lead can come through. Bring your lead hand straight back and collect your opponent's lead hand as you adopt the checkmate position.

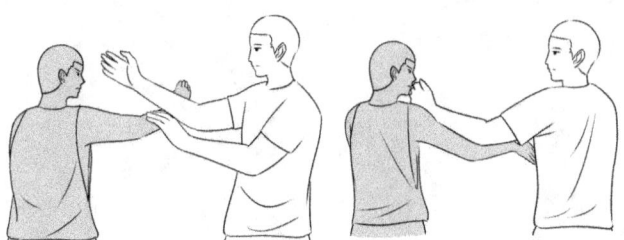

Hammer Entry

With your lead hand slap through your opponent's lower arm and bring it to your rear shoulder.

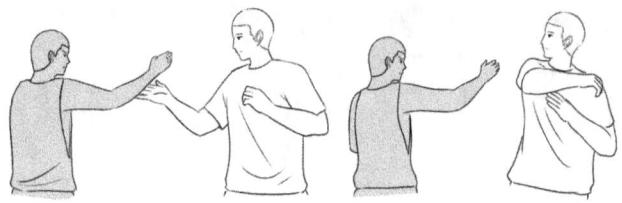

Crash down on your opponent's lead arm with your elbow as your hammer-fist strikes his/her face. Continue moving your lead hand along its path and collect your opponent's lead arm as you move into the checkmate position.

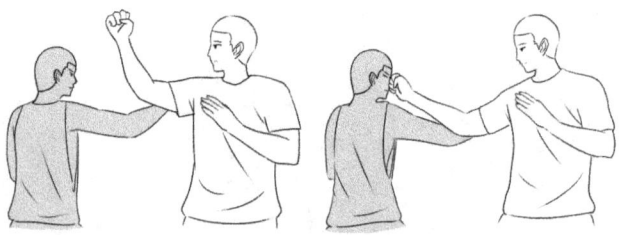

Step Entry

Take a step forward so that you switch your lead side as you close distance with your opponent. As you step forward use your rear hand (which will become the lead) to tap your opponent's lead from the outside, and then bounce off it.

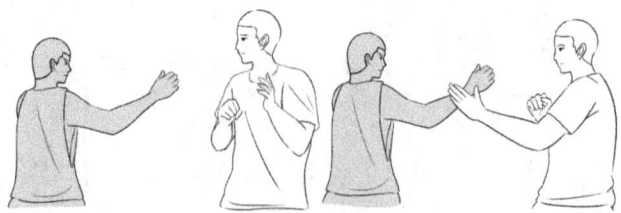

Almost instantaneously, use your other hand (your new rear) to take control of your opponent's lead as you adopt the checkmate position.

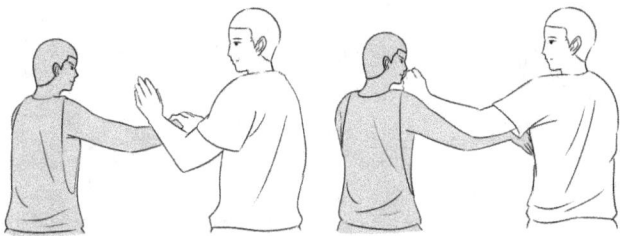

Elbow Entry

Your opponent may strike at you with his/her lead. Cover it with an inside parry. This is more of a backup action, and may not even connect.

As you do the parry, bring your lead elbow up on a vertical plane so that it deflects your opponent's arm to the outside of your body.

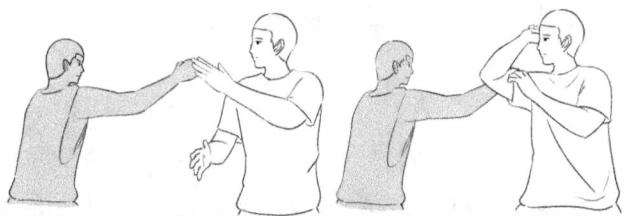

Come down on your opponent's lead with your lead. Do it hard, to hurt his/her arm. Use your rear hand to take control of his/her arm while striking with your lead.

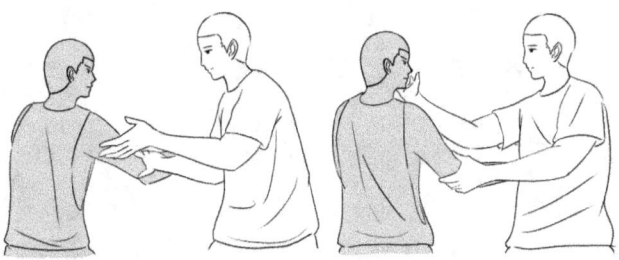

Take control of your opponent's lead with your lead and attack his/her ribs with your rear. Adopt the checkmate position.

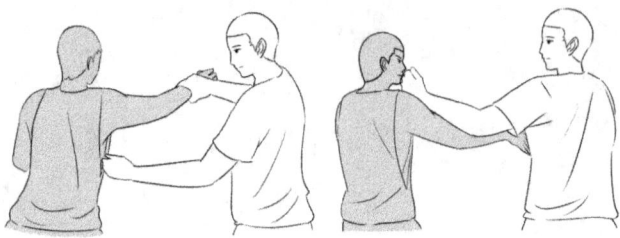

Alternatively, after step two (bringing your elbow up), you can drive your elbow forward into your opponent.

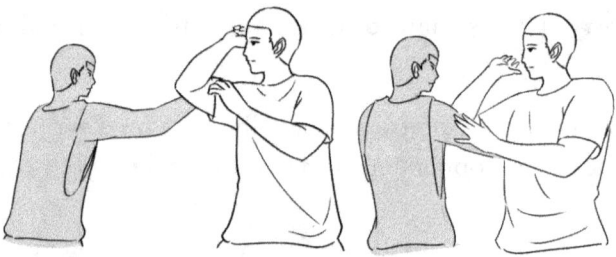

Hook Entry

The hook entry is a big strike entry that uses the hooking strike, as demonstrated in the weight distribution drill.

From the start position, let your lead drop and use your rear to guard your opponent's lead.

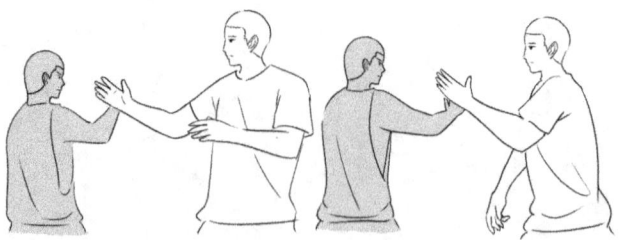

Move your opponent's lead down as you strike through him/her with your lead.

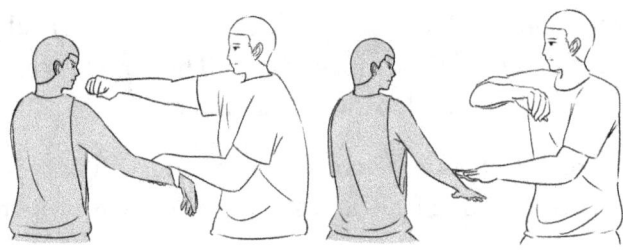

After doing the hook entry, you'll most likely go straight into the hand formula as opposed to checkmate.

Related Chapters:

- Weight Distribution Drill
- Hand Formula

THRUST ENTRIES

Thrust entries are used when your opponent is keeping his/her guard too close to his/her own body (below 120°). The thrust entry collapses your opponent's lead hand in towards him/her.

Most of these thrust entry demonstrations start with both fighters in a right lead stance. Their lead hands are held out wrist-on-wrist.

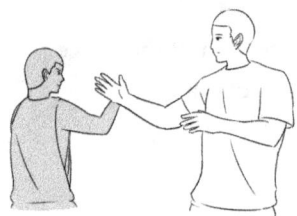

Push Entry

As you step forward, use your rear arm to apply pressure on your opponent's lead arm to clear the centerline. At the same time, strike with your lead.

The best place to apply the pressure is on the forearm, closer to your opponent's elbow. If you're too close to the wrist, your opponent may be able to strike you with his/her elbow.

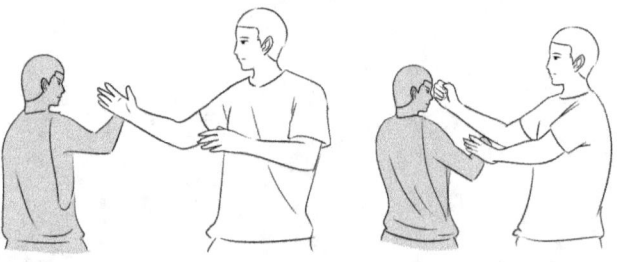

Bring your lead hand straight back and collect your opponent's lead hand as you adopt the checkmate position.

Neck Attack Entry

With the neck attack entry, you drive your lead forearm into your opponent's neck.

As you move forward, use your rear hand to clear the centerline by applying pressure to your opponent's lead arm. Target his/her upper arm/shoulder. Apply the pressure on a "rolling angle" across his/her body and slightly back towards yourself.

At the same time, attack your opponent's neck on an upward angle with your forearm. As your forearm comes into contact with your target, you can give it a little forward torque.

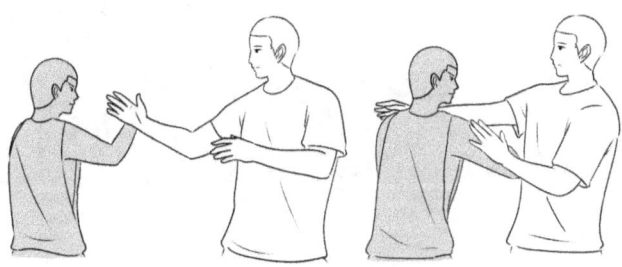

From there, move into the checkmate position.

For a less brutal strike, aim for the chest as opposed to the neck.

When you perform this move, it's important for you to stay grounded. Even when your opponent is slightly taller than you, it is possible. Don't come up on your toes. Instead, ground your left side more and extend the right side your torso.

If needed you can double up on your attack. This may be useful if your first strike missed your target, and/or if your opponent is attempting to grab your arm.

Sink your weight and drop your arm. Sinking your weight resets your spring. Dropping your arm will clear (and hurt) your opponent's arms while creating space for you to repeat your attack.

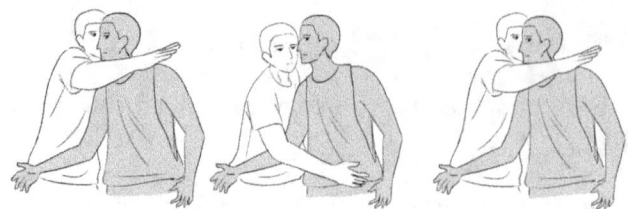

The Push-Neck Combination

The push-neck combination is the push entry immediately followed by the neck attack entry. It's a good demonstration of how entries can flow from one to another.

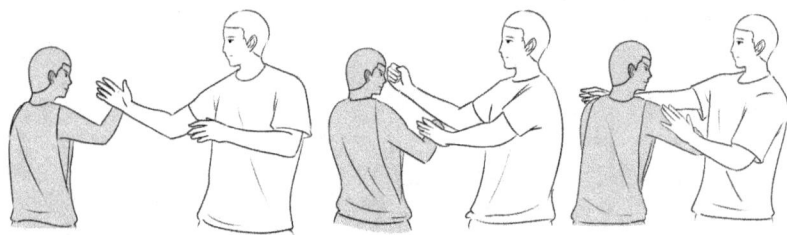

CURVE ENTRIES

Curve entries go around your opponent's guard in some way. When making one, be careful not to open yourself up. Stick to his/her arm, or as close to him/her as you can.

Curve-In Entry

Curl your lead hand around your opponent's, towards the inside of his/her guard. Next, use your rear hand to quickly guard his/her lead as you strike with your lead.

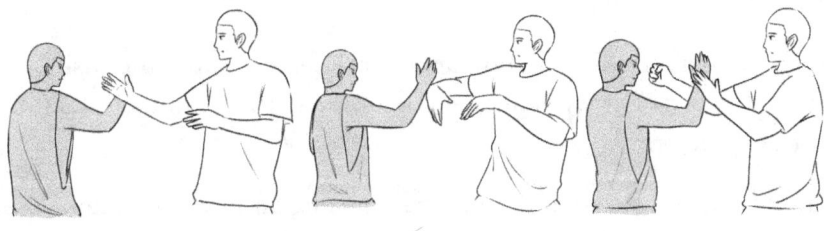

Collect your opponent's lead with your lead and strike with your rear to adopt the checkmate position.

Tap-Curve Entry

Move into the starting position with a slight tap to your opponent's hand and then quickly withdraw.

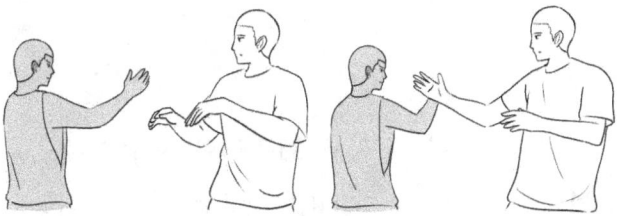

The act of tapping your opponent's hand from one side will cause him/her to resist. It is a feint.

Your opponent's opposing movement leaves his/her centerline open. Strike, and then adopt the checkmate position.

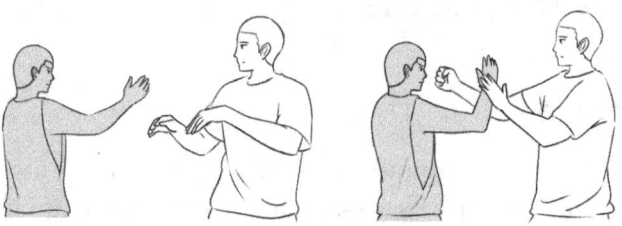

Curve-Under Entry

Curl your hand around your opponent's lead towards the inside of his/her guard. This is done using a more vertical movement than in the curve-in entry.

Lean back and strike from underneath using an upward motion. Use your rear hand to guard your opponent's lead. Adopt the checkmate position.

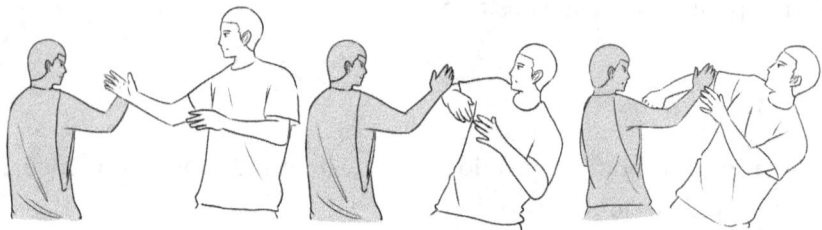

Groin Entry

The groin entry is useful for moving past your opponent.

Step in and use your rear hand to guide your opponent's elbow past you.

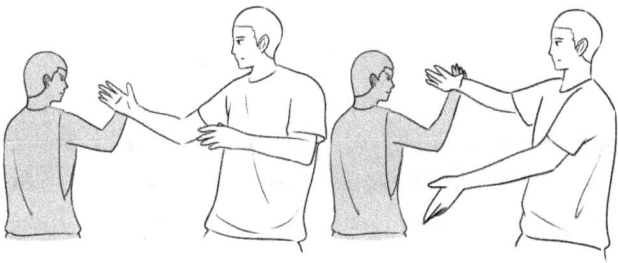

Curve your lead down to attack your opponent's groin.

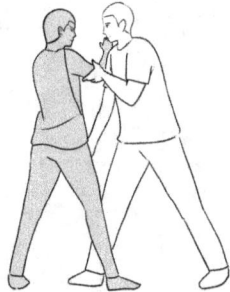

If you're not moving past your opponent, you can go into the checkmate position by bringing your rear hand up the outside of your opponent's guard and then using it to pull his/her lead towards you.

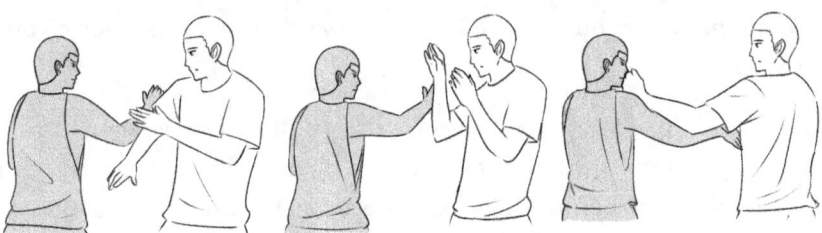

CONTACT ENTRIES

When using a contact entry, you grab hold of your opponent's limb to shift it out of your way. The type of contact entry you use depends on the direction of the pressure (or lack of it) applied by your opponent.

Grab Contact Entry

When your opponent applies forward pressure. flow with it by grabbing his/her arm and moving directly into checkmate.

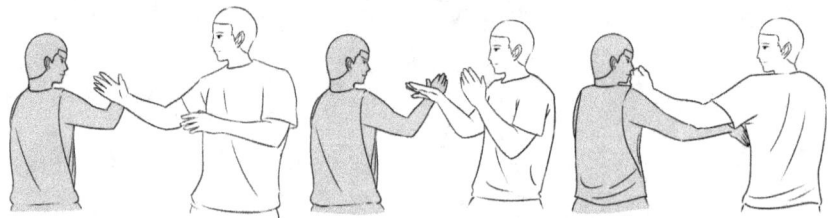

Hook Contact Entry

Use a big rear hooking strike while you pull your opponent in with your lead. Rotate your arm at the shoulder to gain tremendous momentum. As you bring it around toward your target, hook your arm in.

Training Tip: To get the feeling for the pulling-in movement during training, you can get a bit of a wind-up by making small circles with your lead wrist before doing the grab. Use the waterfall action to move over and grab your opponent's wrist.

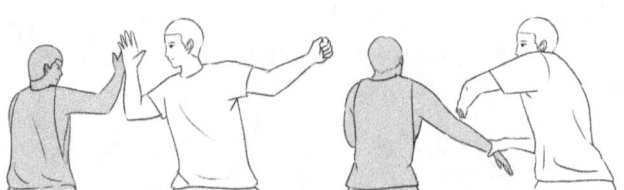

Bring your lead arm back to collect your opponent's arm, twisting him/her back in the opposite direction as you strike with a lead hook.

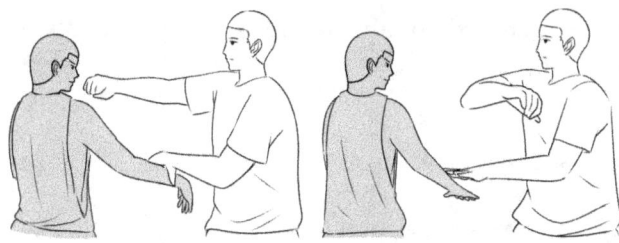

From this position, either continue with the hand formula or go into checkmate.

Push Contact Entry

Use this type of contact entry when your opponent is releasing pressure towards him/herself. Take advantage and pin his/her lead with yours as you strike, then adopt a variation of checkmate.

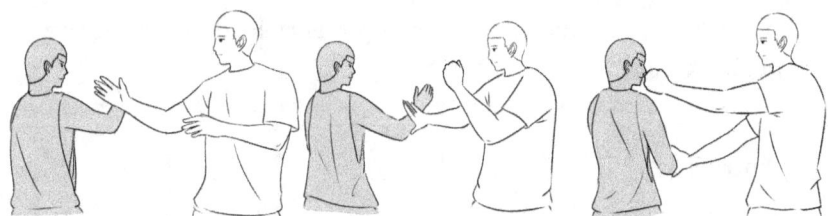

Related Chapters:

- Hand Formula

RIB ENTRIES

The main characteristic of a rib entry is that you attack your opponent's ribs.

Rib Entry One

Bring your lead over your opponent's.

At the same time, use your rear hand to guide your opponent's lead to the outside of your guard as you strike his/her ribs.

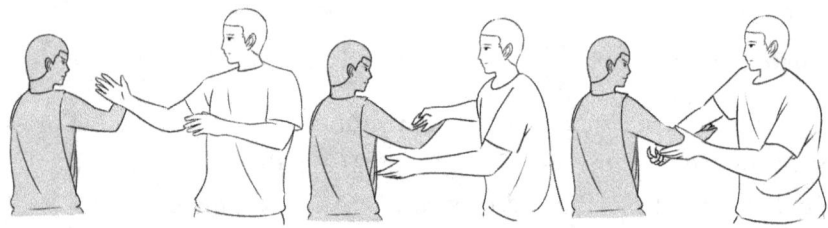

Pull your lead back and grab your opponent's lead along the way to adopt checkmate.

Rib Entry Two

Curl your wrist around your opponent's in the same manner as in the first curve entry.

Guard your opponent's lead with your rear as you strike his/her ribs.

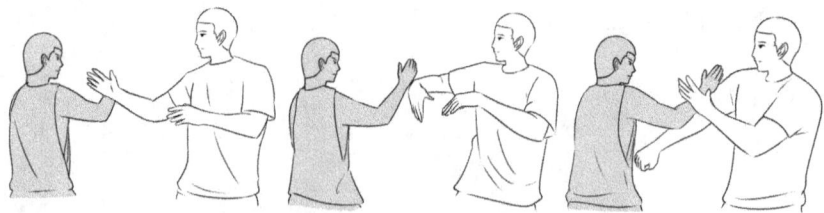

Rib Entry Three

Use your lead hand to guide your opponent's lead towards you.

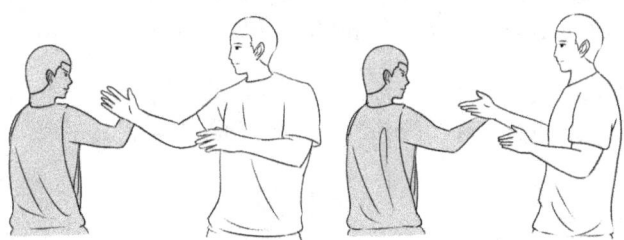

Once your opponent's lead has been extended far enough, use your rear hand to guard his/her lead from behind as you strike the ribs.

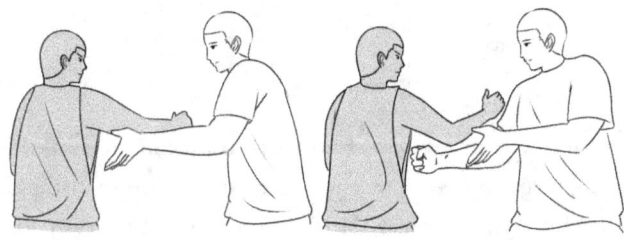

In variations two and three, adopt checkmate by bringing your rear hand up the outside of your opponent's guard and using it to pull his/her lead.

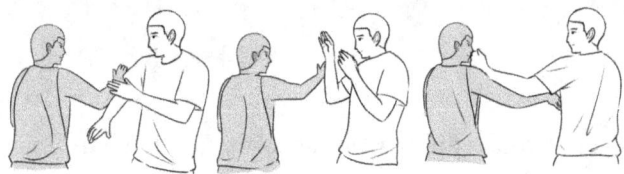

Related Chapters:

- Curve Entries

HAND FORMULA

Once you have completed your entry and achieved the checkmate position you can go into the hand formula described in this section.

From the checkmate position, take control of your opponent's lead arm with your rear hand and twist his/her body as you hook with your lead.

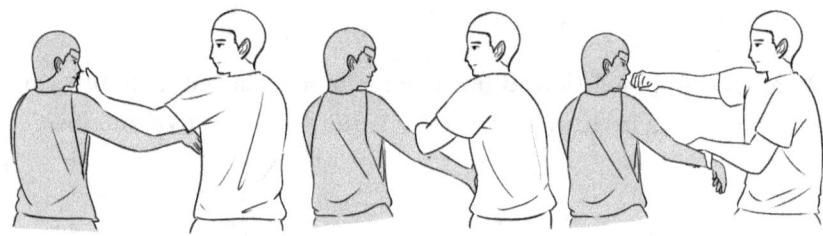

If your opponent puts his/her hand up to block the hook, curl your wrist down to guide it out of the way. Finish the curling circle and continue the hooking motion. This should be one fluid movement.

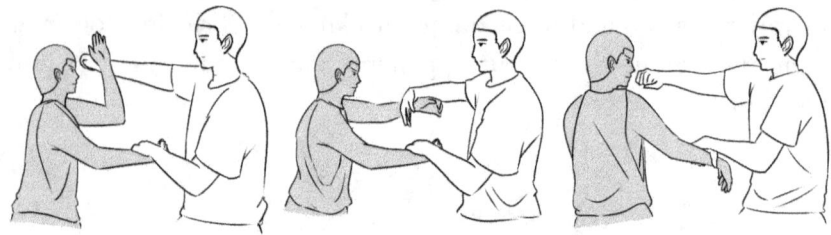

Take control of your opponent's lead with your lead and twist his/her body back the other way. Attack your opponent's ribs.

Use both your hands to jerk your opponent's lead arm down. Drop your weight into it to create a whiplash effect.

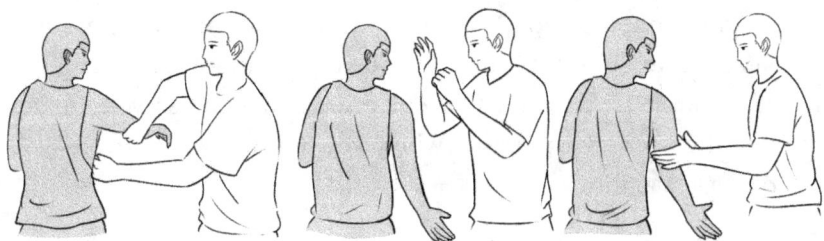

Immediately after pulling your opponent down, bring your lead hand back up to strike him/her underneath the jaw.

Pull your opponent's rear shoulder as you push on his/her lead upper arm to twist him/her back towards you.

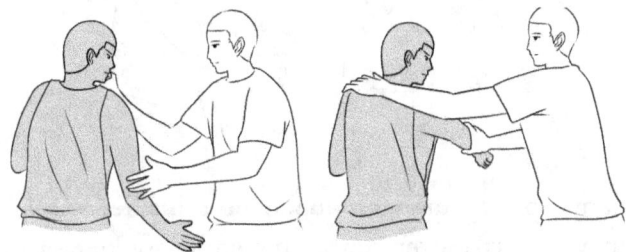

Bring your opponent to his/her knees by simultaneously applying pressure on his/her supra-scapular nerve and using the heel of your foot to push down and forward on the top of his/her calf, just below the knee. How exactly you do this will depend on your angle in relation to your opponent.

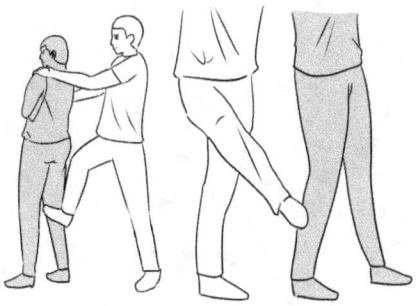

The picture on the left (below) shows the location of the supra-scapular nerve. You don't have to be very accurate when applying pressure point techniques. Just dig in, rub, and press your fingers around the area. You'll know when you hit something from your opponent's reaction.

Chop down on your opponent's supra-scapular nerve and then cup your hands and clap them on your opponent's ears. That is, press his/her head in between your hands.

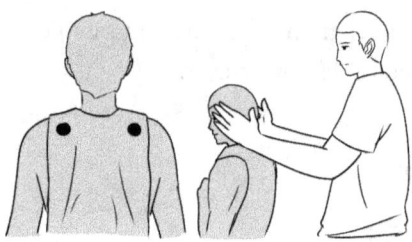

An alternative to bringing your opponent to his/her knees is to do a big hammer-fist strike over your opponent's shoulder. His/her solar plexus is the ideal target.

Apply a choke hold by circling your arms around your opponent's neck and then squeezing them together. Wrap your left arm around the front of your opponent's neck and grab your right elbow. With your right hand along the back of your opponent's neck, grab your left elbow.

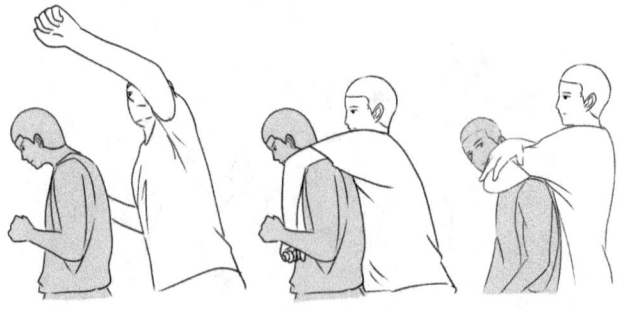

This choke could also be applied once your opponent is on his/her knees.

It's important to know that you don't have to get to checkmate before starting the formula, and in a real fight, you probably won't need to go through the whole formula. Often, just the entry will be enough to finish a fight.

Furthermore, you need not perform the parts of the formula in order. All the elements of Vortex Control Self-Defense, like any martial art, can (and should) be intertwined and used as appropriate for the circumstance and according do your opponent's reaction(s).

Here are just a few of the uncountable variations that you may choose to use:

After attacking the ribs, move directly into attacking your opponent's back.

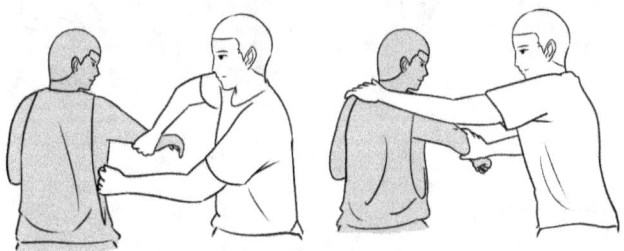

After the hammer entry, move directly into arm pulling.

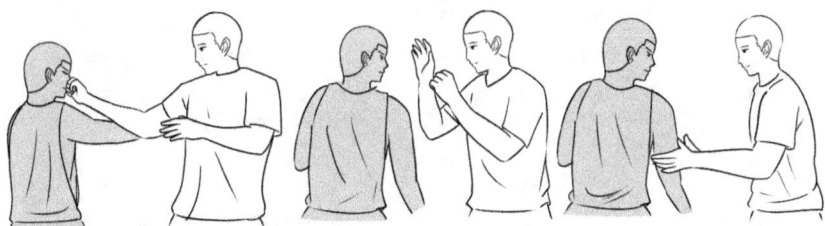

Move back into check-mate after attacking your opponent's ribs. You can repeat this move multiple times.

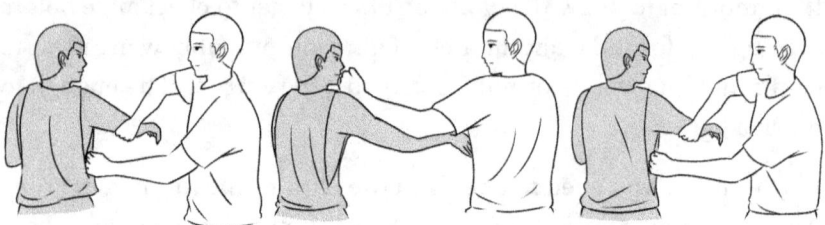

After the hook, move into an underarm pressure lock.

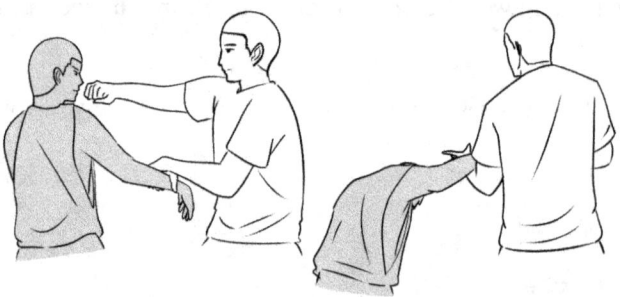

Related Chapters:

- Lock Flow Drill

LOCK FLOW DRILL

The purpose of the lock-flow drill is to teach a wide variety of arm-locks. The term arm-lock encompasses the shoulder, wrist, fingers, etc.

In a self-defense situation, these locks can be used individually or in small combinations to serve your purpose.

Some reasons you may want to apply an arm lock are to:

- Gain pain compliance (to escort somebody out of a room, for example).
- Break an opponent's limb, which is likely to end the conflict.
- Disarm an armed assailant.

When practicing the following lock-flow drill, keep these points in mind:

- As you flow from lock to lock, always have at least one hand griping your opponent's limb. This helps to keep him/her from escaping.
- You can slide your hands along your opponent's limb while still keeping your grip. You'll get better at this with practice.
- Where possible, keep your elbows close to your body. This will enable you to best use your center of gravity to generate power.
- Jerking, vibrating, strikes, etc., can be used to soften your opponent up, making it easier to apply the locks effectively, and/or to increase the damage done. Some examples of these things are included in this chapter's demonstrations.

For ease of remembering and writing, the following locks have been given semi-descriptive, unofficial names.

Shoulder Lock

From the checkmate position, use your left hand to move your opponent's right hand down. At the same time, move your right hand towards your opponent's left shoulder.

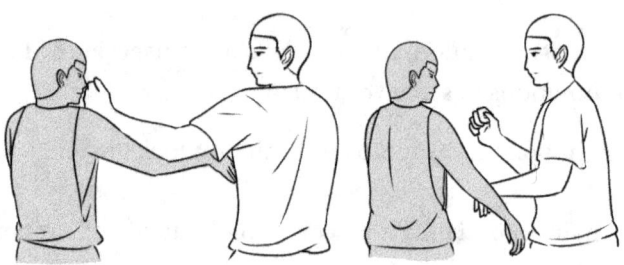

Move your left arm under your opponent's arm to his/her rear, so that the underside of your elbow, which is facing up, can hook onto his/her arm. Bend your opponent forwards by applying pressure on his/her shoulder with your right hand.

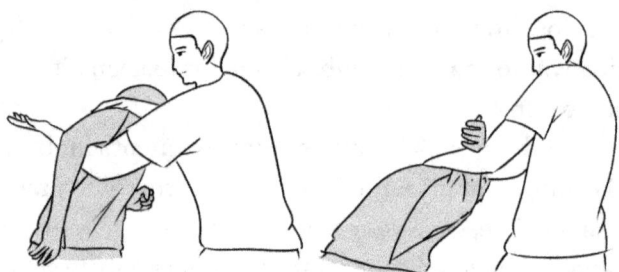

Here, the shoulder lock is shown from the opposite side, and aggression is added.

With the hand that isn't hooking your opponent's arm, strike his/her face on the way to grabbing his/her neck. As you come back to grab your opponent's neck, do so forcefully, using a cupped hand.

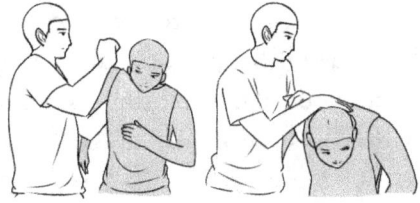

Follow up with another elbow to your opponent's head. You can repeat these two strikes, You can also knee him/her.

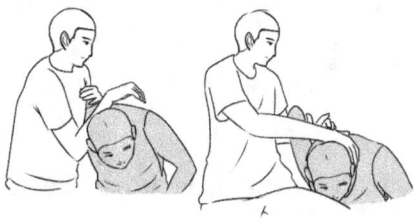

Wrist Twist

Slide your right hand down your opponent's arm to control his/her elbow. At the same time, slide your left hand down and grip at your opponent's wrist.

Your left hand should be on the inside of your opponent's guard, with your palm facing out. Grip your opponent's wrist and then pull his/her arm across your centerline. You can use your right hand to help with a push at your opponent's elbow, although this is usually not needed.

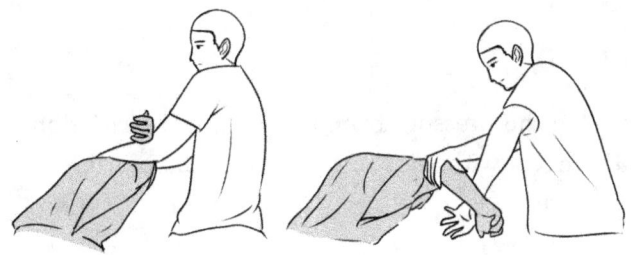

As you bring your opponent's arm across your centerline, continue to slide your right hand down his/her arm to meet your left hand at his/her wrist. Use both your hands to bring your opponent's hand up and then over to the outside of his/her guard. Use the waterfall principle.

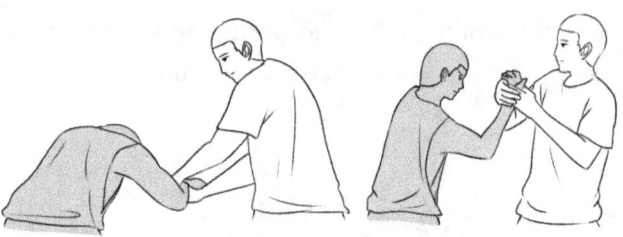

When the wrist twist is fully applied, it has the potential to damage the whole limb.

Wrist Twist Variation

Release the pressure and then apply a variation of the wrist twist by pushing your opponent's wrist down towards him/her.

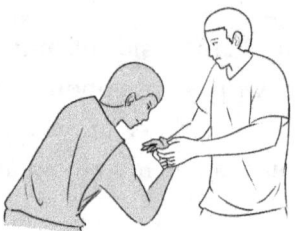

Wrist Lock

As you release the pressure from the wrist twist variation, grip your opponent's fingers with your right hand. Push your opponent's hand into his/her face.

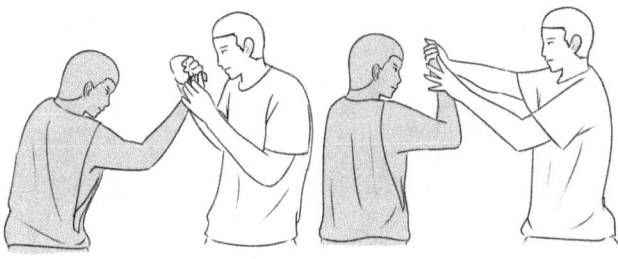

Move your left hand to your opponent's elbow. Push your opponent's elbow as you pull his/her fingers down and towards your centerline.

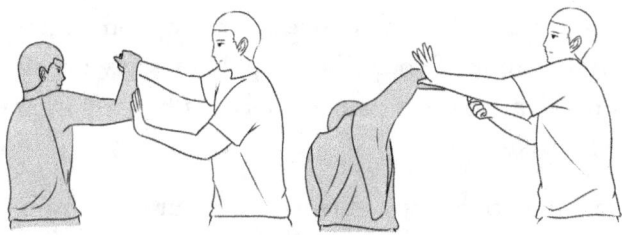

As your opponent's arm straightens, grab hold of his/her thumb with your left hand and then pull his/her hand towards your center. Lock your elbows close to your body and apply torque his/her hand, applying pressure (creating a vortex), to perform the wrist lock.

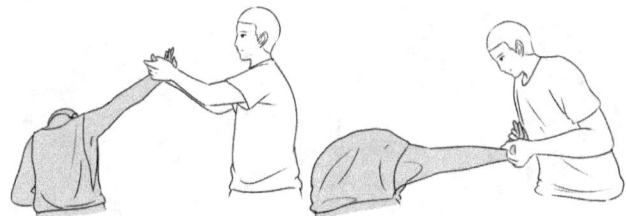

Wrist Pressure

Keep a good grip on your opponent's thumb with your left hand while sliding your right hand up to his/her elbow. Bend his/her arm down vertically at the elbow and use a circular motion to move it to the inside and up.

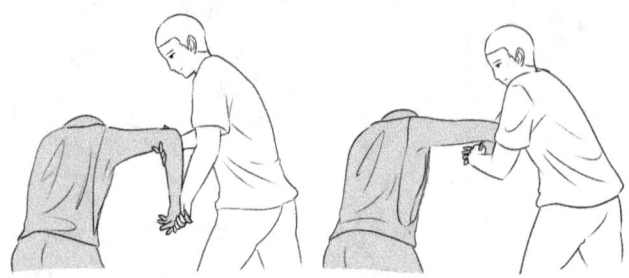

Use your right hand to help place your opponent's upper arm securely in the crook of your elbow. Apply pressure on his/her wrist with your left hand to cause pain and lock his/her arm in. You can use your right to strike.

The image on the right shows the wrist pressure lock from the opposite side. It also shows that you can put your opponent's elbow either on your bicep or your chest. Putting it on your chest is more secure.

Instead of striking, you can also use your spare hand to increase the pressure on your opponent's wrist.

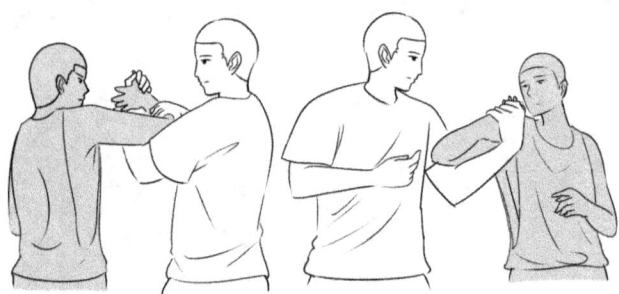

Overarm Pressure

Grip your opponent's wrist with your right hand and then curl your left arm underneath his/hers. At the same time, pull his/her arm straight with your right hand.

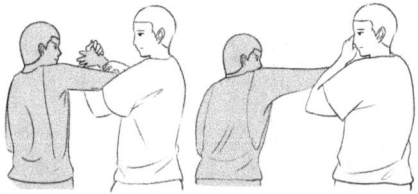

The end result will be that your opponent's arm is straight and his/her elbow faces up. Apply pressure on his/her elbow with your forearm.

As you apply pressure down with your left, pull up with your right. At the same time, use a waterfall motion by applying pressure with your forearm as you roll it over your opponent's elbow.

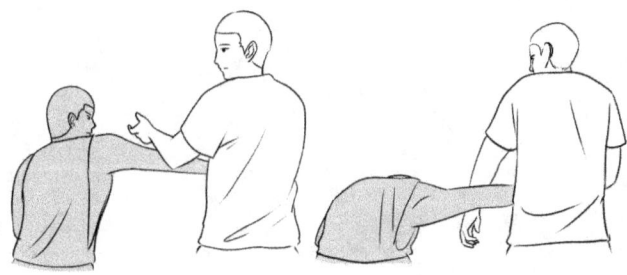

Here it is from the opposite side. You can see the waterfall action more clearly.

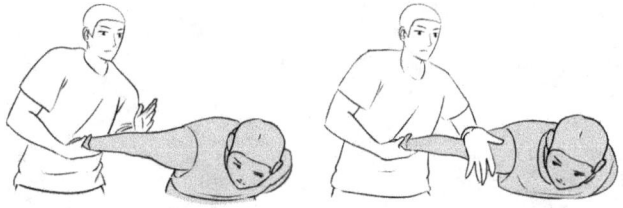

Underarm Pressure

Curl your left slightly toward yourself and then underneath your opponent's arm.

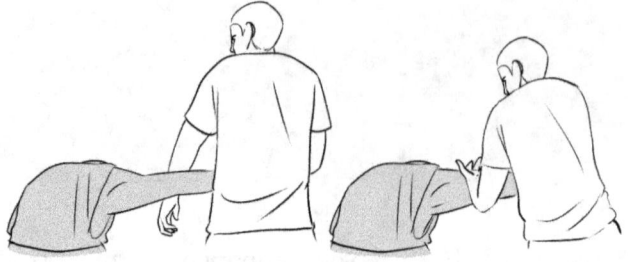

As you do this, your opponent's arm is rolled so that his/her elbow faces the ground.

You apply upward pressure on your opponent's elbow with your own elbow. Your left palm faces up. Apply downward pressure on his/her hand with your right hand.

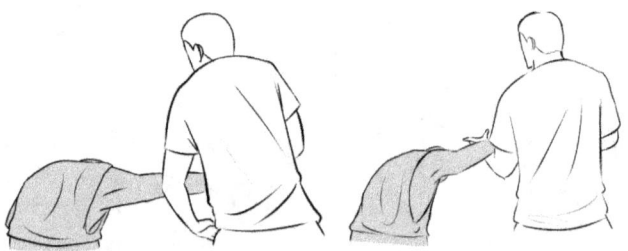

Here it is from the opposite side.

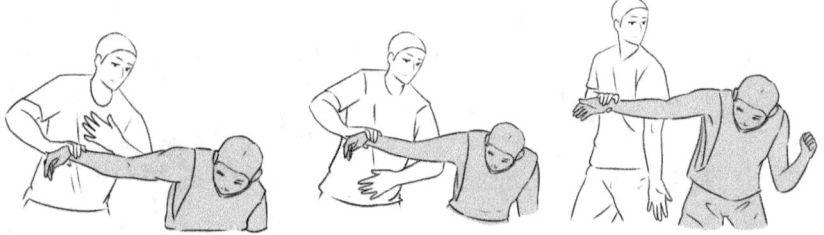

Bent Arm Lock

Return to the overarm pressure lock and then, without letting go of your right hand, bend your opponent's arm towards him/her and grab your right wrist with your left hand. Strike your opponent with your right elbow.

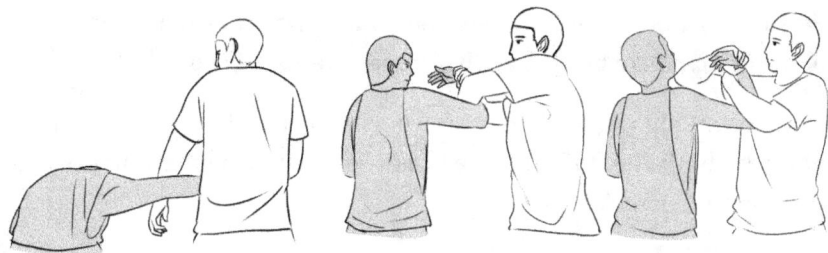

Here it is from the opposite side. Once your arm is on top, you can strike at your opponent's eyes before bending his/her arm.

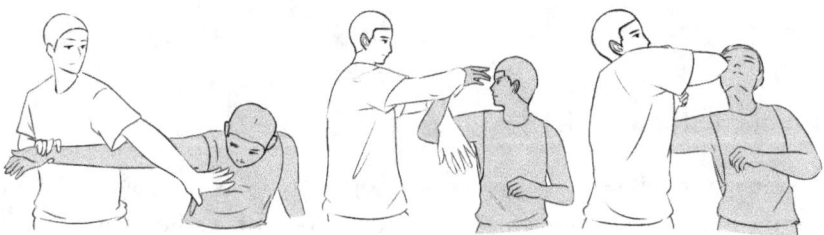

One-Handed Bent Arm Lock

Let go of your right wrist and grab your opponent's fingers from the side facing towards you, so that your palm faces your opponent. Now you have control of your opponent's limb with your left hand.

Move his/her arm away from you and to the outside of his/her shoulder. You can strike him/her with your right hand.

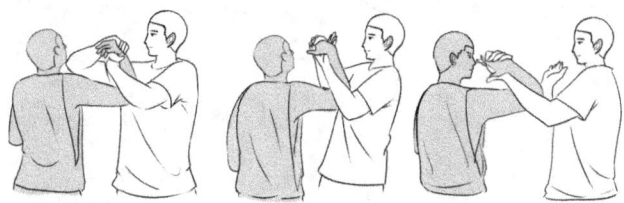

Reverse One-Handed Bent Arm Lock

Bring your right hand up on the outside of your opponent's right arm. Pass it up through the gap between your opponent's wrist and shoulder, and then take hold of his/her fingers, replacing your left hand.

Grab your opponent's hair with your right hand and pull him/her down by both the hair and the wrist. You can also stomp the rear of your opponent's knee.

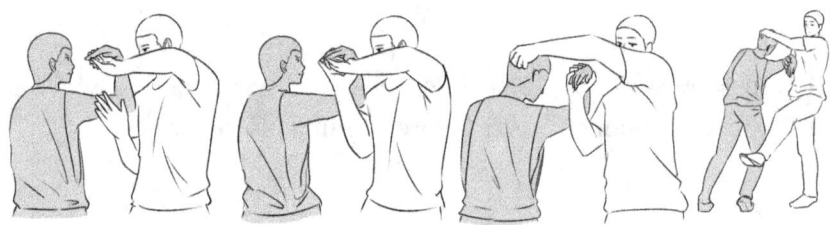

Crooked Elbow Lock

Swing your left arm between your opponent's wrist and shoulder until the crook of your elbow is on the crook of his/her elbow, with your palm facing up. As you do this, release your right hand and catch his/her wrist under your armpit. Apply upward pressure with your left arm.

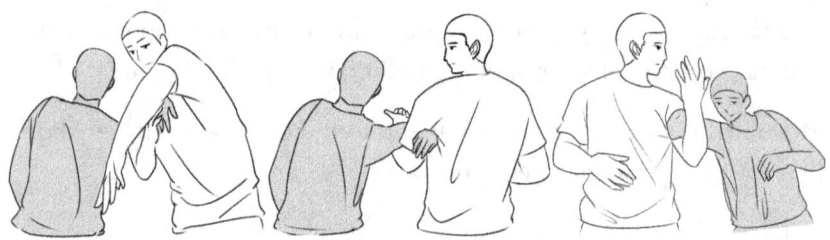

Over-Shoulder Arm Bar

Reach over with your right arm, grab your opponent's left wrist, and pull it towards you. Pass it across your opponent's body, in between his/her body and your left hand.

Place your right hand on the back of your opponent's left shoulder and your left hand on his/her lower left arm, twisting his/her body towards your left shoulder.

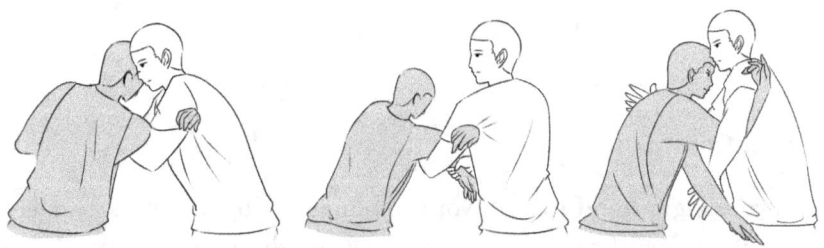

Drop your left arm and use it to attack your opponent's neck. The twist-and-strike action should occur very quickly so you can use the momentum it creates to put more force behind the strike.

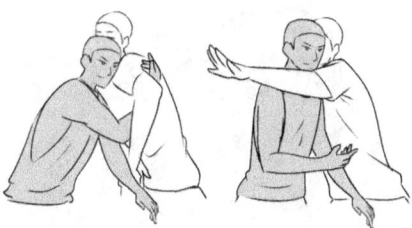

Turn your body so that you're facing the same way as your opponent. At the same time, drop both your hands to grab his/her left hand.

When you drop your hands, be sure to keep your opponent's arm between them. Grab your opponent's wrist with your left hand and take hold of his/her fingers with your right.

Continue to turn your body to the left as you straighten your opponent's arm over your shoulder. His/her elbow should sit on your shoulder, with the underside of the elbow facing up. Pull down on your opponent's wrist to apply pressure.

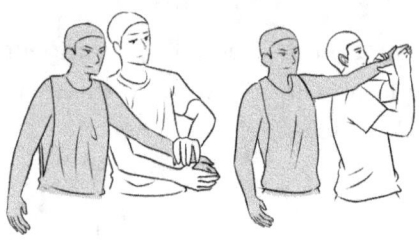

Finger Control

Use your right hand to grab your opponent's ring and pinky fingers. Bend those two fingers down back towards him/her. As you do so, bring his/her lower arm down so that it's aligned along the top of yours. Keep your left hand on his/her wrist.

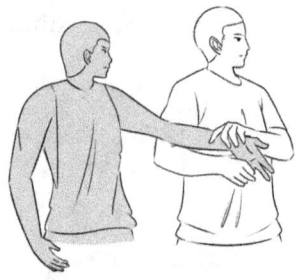

Begin to spin your opponent, so that you swap sides. Do so initially by bending his/her fingers back as you apply pressure on his/her left arm with your right arm.

Keep your opponent's hand near your waist for better leverage on his/her fingers. Pain compliance will keep him/her spinning once your lower arms lose contact.

Finger Lock

Towards the end of the spin, as your opponent is still spinning, use your left hand to grab his/her index and middle fingers.

The third image below shows the finger grab from the opposite side.

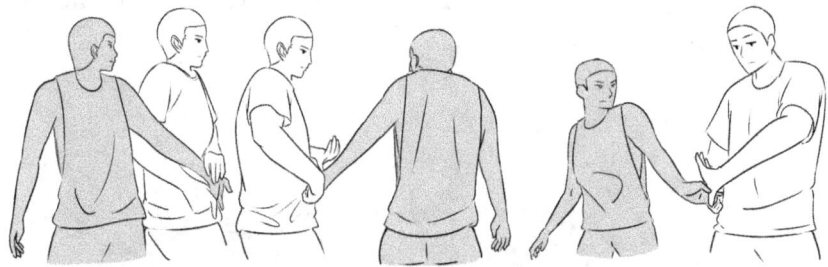

Keeping your opponent's arm straight, bring his/her hand up with his/her bent fingers pointing up. Jerk your opponent's hand down towards you.

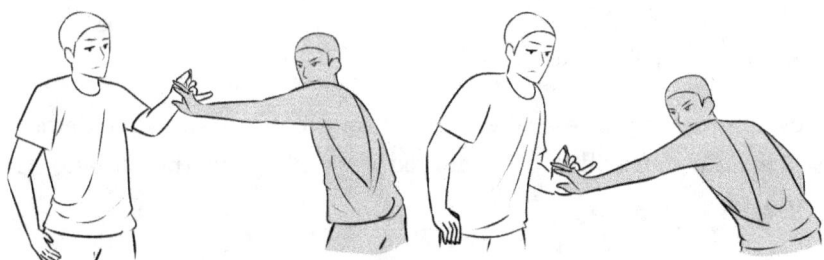

Forearm Torque

Bring your right arm, with your palm facing up, under your opponent's left arm. Place the crook of your elbow just above your opponent's elbow.

Grab your opponent's right wrist with your right hand. Pull his/her hand down by the wrist while applying pressure on his/her elbow with your right arm.

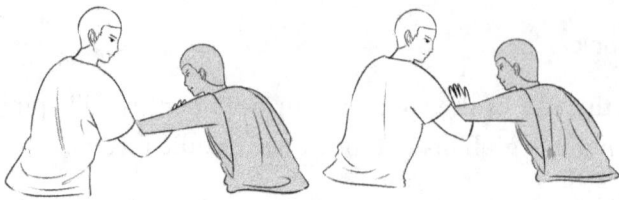

At this point your opponent's forearm should be vertical, with his/her elbow pointing upward, while his/her upper arm should be horizontal.

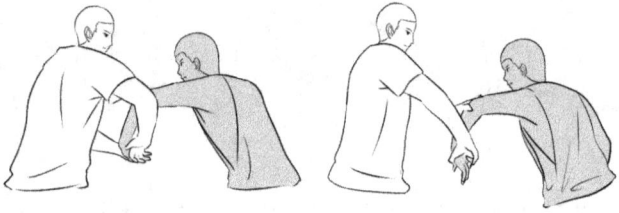

This completes the basic lock-flow drill.

Lock-Flow Drill Alternatives

Now a few (of countless) alternative movements are shown to demonstrate how the drill can be altered depending on the situation at hand.

Wrist-Twist Alternative

This demonstrates how you can go back to the formula from the lock-flow drill. It also shows how you can flow from the rib entry to an upward chin strike as opposed to going to checkmate and then the formula.

At the end of the wrist twist, release the pressure on your opponent's wrist and strike him/her in the ribs, as you would in the rib entry.

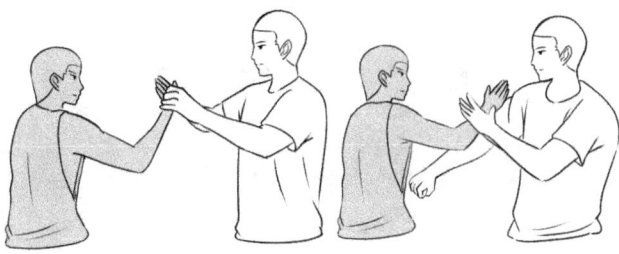

Continue with the rib entry as normal by bringing your hand up to the outside of your opponent's guard.

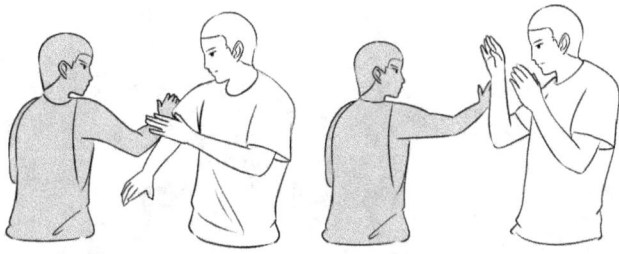

Instead of going into checkmate, you can go straight into the arm pull, and follow it with an upward palm heel to your opponent's jaw.

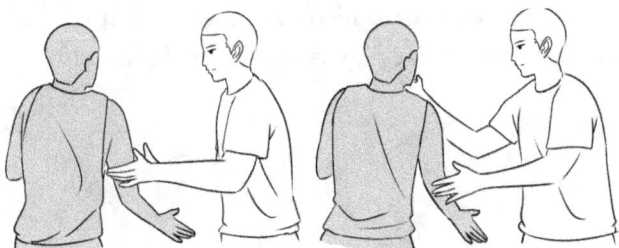

Crooked Elbow Lock to Figure-4 Arm-bar

After you release the pressure from the crooked elbow lock, it's possible for your opponent to swing at you. Use a variation of the elbow entry to block the attack. For example, raise your right elbow.

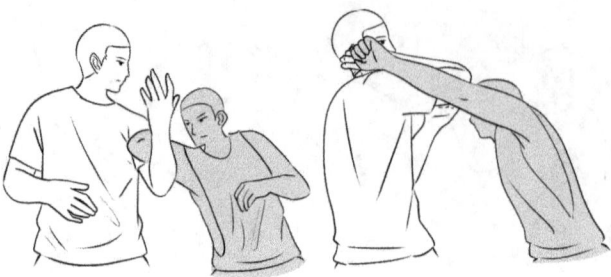

Capture your opponent's arm by circling your right arm over his/her left arm. At the same time place your left hand on your opponent's right shoulder.

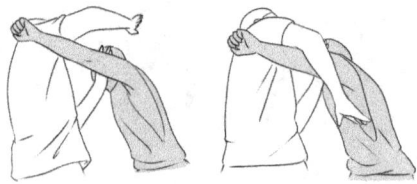

Grab your left forearm with your right hand. Your opponent's straight arm should be in the crook of your right elbow. Apply the figure-4 arm-bar by pushing down on your opponent's shoulder while applying upward pressure on his/her elbow. As you release the lock, strike your opponent's solar plexus with your right hand.

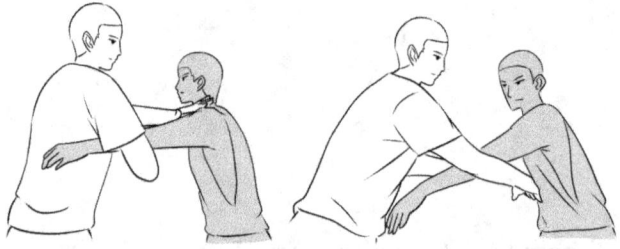

Slide your left hand down your opponent's left arm and grab hold of his/her wrist. As you do this, give him/her a right hook to the jaw. Continue into the over-shoulder arm bar.

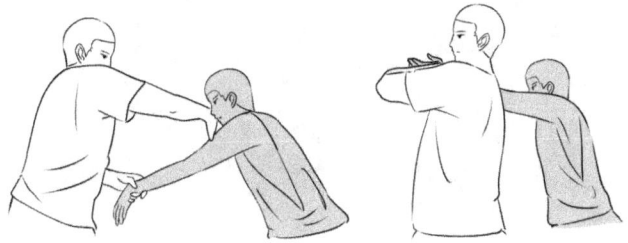

Alternative Ending

This demonstration gives a different ending to the lock flow drill. It starts from the finger lock. Bring your opponent's fingers up to the right side of your chest. With your left hand deliver an uppercut underneath your opponent's left arm to his/her jaw.

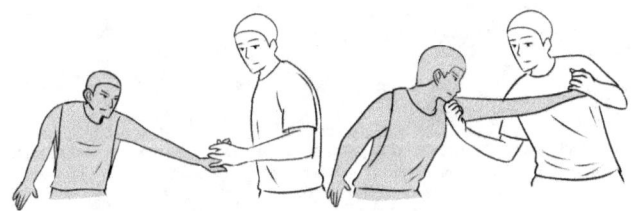

Use your right hand to control the back of your opponent's head so you can bend his/her left arm behind and down his/her back. You'll need to adjust the grip of your left hand to do so.

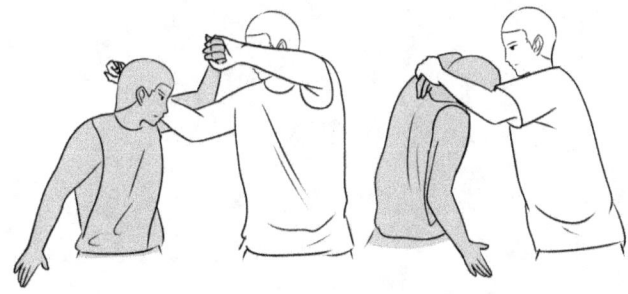

Bring your right hand up underneath your opponent's right armpit and grab his/her left hand. Use your right hand to help force it down. You can release your left hand.

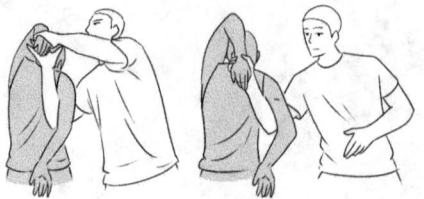

Related Chapters:

- Rib Entries

THANKS FOR READING

Dear reader,

Thank you for reading *Vortex Control Self-Defense*.

If you enjoyed this book, please leave a review where you bought it. It helps more than most people think.

Don't forget your FREE book chapters!

You will also be among the first to know of FREE review copies, discount offers, bonus content, and more.

Go to:

https://offers.SFNonfictionBooks.com/Free-Chapters

Thanks again for your support.

REFERENCES

Abenir, F. (2014). *Eskrima Street Defense: Practical Techniques for Dangerous Situations*. Tambuli Media.

Anderson, D. (2013). *De-Fanging The Snake: A Guide To Modern Arnis Disarms*. CreateSpace Independent Publishing Platform.

Anderson, D. (2013). *Filipino Martial Arts - The Core Basics, Structure, & Essentials*. CreateSpace Independent Publishing Platform.

Anderson, D. (2014). *Trankada: The Joint Locking Techniques & Tapi-Tapi of Modern Arnis*. CreateSpace Independent Publishing Platform.

Cheung, W. (1852). *Dynamic Chi Sao by William Cheung*. Unique Publications.

DeMile, J. (1977). *Tao of Wing Chun Do, Vol. 2: Bruce Lee's Chi Sao*. Tao of Wing Chun Do.

Godhania, K. (2012). *Eskrima: Filipino Martial Art*. Crowood.

Gould, D. (2016). *Lameco Eskrima: The Legacy of Edgar G. Sulite*. Tambuli Media.

Gutierrez, V. (2009). *WingTsun. Chi Sao II*. Sportimex.

Medina, D. (2014). *The Secret Art of Derobio Escrima: Martial Art of the Philippines*. Tambuli Media.

Paman, J. (2007). *Arnis Self-Defense: Stick, Blade, and Empty-Hand Combat Techniques of the Philippines*. Blue Snake Books.

Wiley, M. (2015). *Mastering Eskrima Disarms*. Tambuli Media.

Yimm Lee, J. (1972). *Wing Chun Kung-Fu*. Ohara Publications.

AUTHOR RECOMMENDATIONS

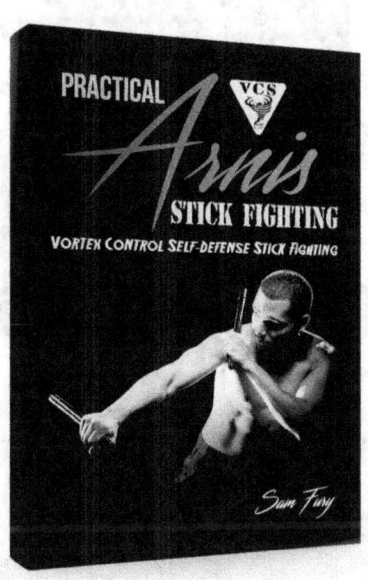

Teach Yourself Stick Fighting for Self-Defense

Teach yourself *Practical Arnis Stick Fighting* today, because the traditional stuff doesn't work on the streets.

Get it now.

www.SFNonfictionBooks.com/Practical-Arnis-Stick-Fighting

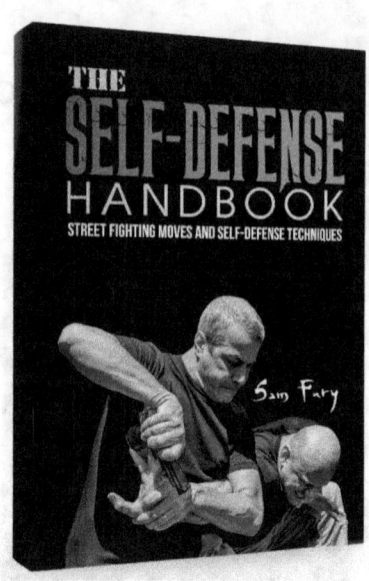

Discover all the Street Fighting Techniques You Need

Start learning what you need to win, because there ain't no rules on the streets.

Get it now.

www.SFNonfictionBooks.com/Self-Defense-Handbook

ABOUT SAM FURY

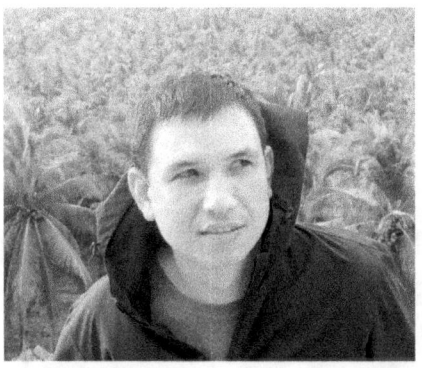

Sam Fury has had a passion for survival, evasion, resistance, and escape (SERE) training since he was a young boy growing up in Australia.

This led him to years of training and career experience in related subjects, including martial arts, military training, survival skills, outdoor sports, and sustainable living.

These days, Sam spends his time refining existing skills, gaining new skills, and sharing what he learns via the Survival Fitness Plan website.

www.SurvivalFitnessPlan.com

- amazon.com/author/samfury
- goodreads.com/SamFury
- facebook.com/AuthorSamFury
- instagram.com/AuthorSamFury
- youtube.com/SurvivalFitnessPlan

www.ingramcontent.com/pod-product-compliance
Lightning Source LLC
Chambersburg PA
CBHW071029080526
44587CB00015B/2546